YOUR KNOWLEDGE HAS VALUE

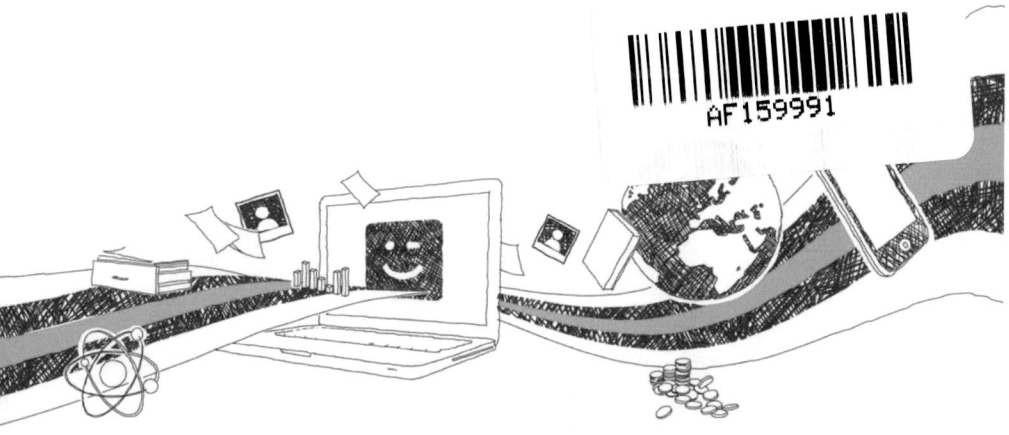

- We will publish your bachelor's and master's thesis, essays and papers

- Your own eBook and book - sold worldwide in all relevant shops

- Earn money with each sale

Upload your text at www.GRIN.com
and publish for free

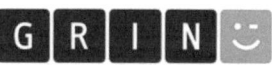

Bibliographic information published by the German National Library:

The German National Library lists this publication in the National Bibliography;
detailed bibliographic data are available on the Internet at http://dnb.dnb.de .

This book is copyright material and must not be copied, reproduced, transferred,
distributed, leased, licensed or publicly performed or used in any way except as
specifically permitted in writing by the publishers, as allowed under the terms and
conditions under which it was purchased or as strictly permitted by applicable
copyright law. Any unauthorized distribution or use of this text may be a direct
infringement of the author s and publisher s rights and those responsible may be
liable in law accordingly.

Imprint:

Copyright © 2018 GRIN Verlag
Print and binding: Books on Demand GmbH, Norderstedt Germany
ISBN: 9783668676138

This book at GRIN:

https://www.grin.com/document/418711

Patrick Kimuyu

The Age-old Practice of Euthanasia

GRIN Verlag

GRIN - Your knowledge has value

Since its foundation in 1998, GRIN has specialized in publishing academic texts by students, college teachers and other academics as e-book and printed book. The website www.grin.com is an ideal platform for presenting term papers, final papers, scientific essays, dissertations and specialist books.

Visit us on the internet:

http://www.grin.com/

http://www.facebook.com/grincom

http://www.twitter.com/grin_com

The Age-old Practice of Euthanasia

Name: Patrick Kimuyu

Table of Contents

Introduction 3
Forms of Euthanasia 4
    Active Euthanasia 4
    Passive Euthanasia 4
    Voluntary Euthanasia 5
    Involuntary Euthanasia 5
    Indirect Euthanasia 6
    Assisted Euthanasia 6
Euthanasia Ethics 7
Arguments for Euthanasia 8
Arguments against Euthanasia 10
Euthanasia and Religion 10
Legislation on Euthanasia 11
Conclusion 12
References 13

Introduction

Euthanasia is commonly known as mercy killing or assisted suicide because the involved procedures are designed in such a way that, the patient's dignity is not degraded or compromised. The Greeks termed it as *euthanatos* which simply meant easy death (Keown, 2002). It involves termination of an individual's life through painless means such as injecting the patient with a lethal drug or withdrawing supply of essential requirements like food and oxygen (Frost, n.d). It is executed at an individual's consent especially when someone is suffering from an incurable health condition. In addition, the decision to terminate a patient's life can also be made by the patient's relatives, the court of law or medical practitioners. However, it is worth noting that the decision by the relatives, the court or the medics is only reached at if the patient is critically ill, such that he or she cannot think or reason. Some individuals who are not terminally ill can sign consent for their lives to be terminated through euthanasia because of ethical reasons especially with matters related to human dignity, but this happens on rare occasions (Keown, 2002). However, euthanasia has aroused unprecedented debate in the society because it involves several considerations; the most significant one's being practical, religious and ethical issues. Moreover, this practice seems to be somehow challenging to the health professionals, since it is not in alignment with the medical ethics nor legal framework. Euthanasia is illegal in the United Kingdom: thus, it is considered illegal. Therefore, approaches towards euthanasia require caution, since it can lead to imprisonment (Nicholson, 2000). For instance, voluntary euthanasia is considered as a crime in the United Kingdom, which is punishable by law. Any individual who deliberately executes euthanasia is subjected to serve a jail term. Therefore, this research paper will give an overview of euthanasia. Euthanasia has evoked unprecedented controversy in the society.

Forms of Euthanasia

Euthanasia can be performed in various ways, some of which are considered unethical while others are relatively acceptable, although unprecedented controversy looms over the ethics of euthanasia. The forms of euthanasia are categorized according to the nature of the approaches undertaken during the termination of an individual's life. In general, euthanasia can be categorized as either active or passive. This approach is based on the procedure that is adopted in executing one's life. That is, the practitioner's decision on whether to inject the patient with a lethal dose or by withdrawing treatment and letting one die of the disease condition. On the other hand, euthanasia can be categorized according to the patient's decision on his or her death. In this case, euthanasia can be termed as voluntary or involuntary. Moreover, euthanasia can be categorized with respect to approach and wish of either the patient or the medic. In such a scenario, euthanasia is classified as indirect euthanasia or assisted euthanasia.

Active Euthanasia

Ordinarily, active euthanasia involves deliberate killing of the patient through performing a suicidal act that causes the death of the patient (Keown, 2002). For instance, medics may give the patient an overdose of the conventional drugs such as pain-killers, which will ultimately result into a sudden death of the patient. This is a deliberate act because the concerned medics are aware of the outcomes, even though they do not actively kill the patient. This form of euthanasia is morally unacceptable because medics do it out of will, and the drug doses may not reach the intended lethal level (Keown, 2002). In the event that the doses do not cause death to the patient, critical ethical issues can emerge leading to unprecedented ethical problems.

Passive Euthanasia

In passive euthanasia, medics let the patient die on their own by withdrawing essential requirements such treatment, oxygen and food. Withdrawal of treatment to a patient involves termination of treatment approaches such as switching off life-supporting machines (Keown, 2002). As a result, the patient dies of the disease condition because he or she cannot survive without supportive facilities. Withdrawal of treatment may include turning off gas and food supply tubes or termination of medication that are required by the patient to live.

On the other hand, a patient can be killed through withholding of treatment that could have saved that patient's life (Busè, 2008). For instance, patients whose treatment requires surgery of a vital body organ such as the heart or brain can be allowed to die by failing to carry out surgery to extend his or her life. Ordinarily, surgery is believed to extend the lives of patients because it restores the defective body organ or system.

From a moral perspective, passive euthanasia is considered to be more ethical than active euthanasia. However, some people express total objection to it; since it imparts ethical consequences to the relatives of the patient. This is so because; it evokes immense emotions especially when the process does not cause death over a short period.

Voluntary Euthanasia

In voluntary euthanasia, the ailing individuals request to be killed. It also happens if the person who seeks to die prefers to maintain his or her dignity. An old person may request for euthanasia, even if he or she is not terminally ill. In other words, voluntary euthanasia is performed, incase in individual requests for his or her life to be terminated because of ethical reasons, and not necessarily as a result of illness.

Involuntary Euthanasia

Involuntary euthanasia occurs in circumstances in which the person, who is to be killed wishes to live, but other parties, rather than the concerned individual consider it necessary to terminate his or her life because of various reasons. In most cases, involuntary euthanasia is performed on unconscious individuals or in people who are mentally unable to choose between death and life. For instance, individuals with low levels of intelligence such as young babies are unable to comprehend the essence of euthanasia. As a result, euthanasia decision is made on their behalf especially by relatives or medics. However, it is worth noting that such decisions must be in accordance to the law. Ordinarily, involuntary euthanasia is done on infants who are born with fatal biological defects that may not allow the child to survive. In most cases, involuntary euthanasia is performed by soldiers in the battle field when their fellow soldiers sustain fatal injuries that cause severe pain.

Indirect Euthanasia

Indirect euthanasia appears to be relatively different from the other forms of euthanasia because it is performed in a sophisticated approach. In indirect euthanasia, the patient is put on treatment that involves administration of pain-relieving drugs to the patient, which later causes fatal side-effects, leading to the patient's death. The drugs' side effects hasten the death of the patient, even though he or she does not experience the pain caused by the disease condition. This form of euthanasia is known as the doctrine of double effect. It has been found that indirect euthanasia is morally acceptable; since the principal intention is to relieve pain, but not to kill the patient. It is relatively non-intentional, even though it is termed as euthanasia in the medical ethics.

Assisted Euthanasia

Assisted euthanasia is commonly confused with the factual meaning of euthanasia. Contrary to the perception of many people, assisted euthanasia simply implies that the person who wishes to die is provided with suicidal means. For instance, lethal drugs can be made available to the patient who requires assistance to kill themselves, upon request, but the second party does not have any contribution in decision-making or the suicide mission. The patient takes away his or her life through taking the drugs that have been placed within their reach (Foley & Hendin, 2002).

Euthanasia Ethics

Euthanasia ethics seem to have evoked unprecedented controversy in the society. Currently, there are different opinions regarding the ethics of euthanasia and this situation has been worsened by the legal framework of many countries. Some countries do not have efficient legislations that define the precepts of euthanasia, while others have prohibition laws such as the United Kingdom.

It appears that the current debate over euthanasia is seemingly becoming ambiguous because different groups of individuals view it from diverse perspectives. Some individuals consider it to be necessary to assist a terminally ill patient, who is suffering from an incurable health condition to die (Nicholson, 2000). However, it appears somehow difficult to single out the moral differences between euthanasia and normal death because; whether the patient is assisted to die or allowed to get to the eventual normal death, the ultimate result is death. The second moral dilemma that has made euthanasia appear to confuse is the circumstances under which it is suppose to be executed, since there is a total absence of a consensus justification of euthanasia.

Ordinarily, human beings associate life and death with extremely sensitive ethical values and meaning. They hold the notion that life and death are critical aspects of humanity; therefore, they are solely responsible for making decisions regarding these aspects. In contrast, euthanasia seems to be independently related to the fundamental tenets of humanity, leading to the unprecedented debate in the society.

In general, arguments over euthanasia are primarily based on practical, religious and ethical issues. The key factors that compel an individual to seek for euthanasia are pain and psychological factors such as depression. Pain caused by disease conditions becomes relatively unbearable at some disease levels. For instance, patients who experience intense pain and suffering because of some health conditions such as breathlessness, incontinence and paralysis consider an early death than prolonged agony caused by pain and discomfort. Recent survey reports that were conducted in the U.S showed that most patients who request for euthanasia face severe physical conditions, which seem to degrade the quality of life (Nicholson, 2000). Further survey results showed that a third of patients in the Netherlands seek for euthanasia because of severe pain that is caused by their illnesses.

Arguments for Euthanasia

Proponents of euthanasia argue from various perspectives. Most of their arguments are based on practical, philosophical and medical perspectives.

Libertarians argue that people should be allowed to make independent choices over their lives. They believe that death is a private issue, which does not involve other people. Therefore, one can request for euthanasia, as long as, it will not interfere with the lives of other people. Moreover, they argue that conventional human rights leave the decision to die to an individual. They argue that dying is a human right and exceptionally personal. Therefore, the decision to choose whether to die or live lies on the individual. They claim that euthanasia is necessary for someone who considers dying, rather than, experiencing unbearable pain, if it does not cause harm to other people. They vehemently insist that an individual's decision on life do not need to be interfered with, since other people do not rightfully decide over one's life. Secondly, libertarians argue that euthanasia can be regulated through defining circumstances at which it can be sought for, in the event that an individual faces severe health conditions. In addition, they suggest that legitimizing euthanasia will help to reduce the burden on healthcare resources, which are currently strained by high costs of maintaining the terminally ill patients. Therefore, they consider it to be realistic if euthanasia is allowed because it can ensure equitable distribution of healthcare resources. Moreover, philosophers have posed a utilitarian argument that universality on moral rules can be enhanced through euthanasia (Bowie & Bowie, 2004). If euthanasia can be universalized, then death can become an option in one's life: thus, enabling patients who prefer dying than living to receive social justice. They claim that euthanasia is morally acceptable because it is usually done with the consent of the ailing individual, and it does not infringe upon the rights of other people.

From a philosophical approach, euthanasia serves a pivotal role in homogenizing the principal moral rules. Ordinarily, philosophers believe that moral rules exhibit a degree of universality, a criterion that is satisfied by euthanasia.

A utilitarian approach considers death as a necessary phenomenon in the life of a human being; therefore, euthanasia brings the same impacts as natural death. They hold that death is not a dreadful thing because it is an ordinary phenomenon: thus dying is as significant as living.

On the other hand, medics view euthanasia as a reliable medical approach that relieves patients of severe agony and pain. They validate their claim by stating that, even if a patient is allowed to die eventually, death will come at the end after having tormented one's life. In addition, they claim that healthcare is burdened with treatment of terminally ill patients: thus performing euthanasia on such patients can free up healthcare resources. This argument has also been supported by economists and policy planners; since it will reduce the cost of treatment through creating efficient accessibility to healthcare facilities.

Arguments against Euthanasia

On the other hand, opponents of euthanasia seem to express a varied approach to the issue. However, their arguments are extremely diverse because they are based on a number of aspects. These aspects include moral concerns, medical ethics and religious issues.

They argue that euthanasia devalues life because it interferes with the fundamental processes of human life. They claim that death should be perceived as a natural phenomenon like birth and life as a whole. Secondly, opponents of the euthanasia practice argue that it goes against the best interests of the society since individuals hold some degree of value and meaning in the society. Therefore, allowing euthanasia appears to impart elements of fear into someone's life. Thirdly, opponents of euthanasia have raised fears over the regulation of the issue, since it may compromise medical ethics. For instance, approval of euthanasia as part of the medical procedures may compromise the performance of healthcare professionals. Fourthly, they argue that promoting universality of euthanasia may introduce pressure and abuse (Dobson & Galbraith, 2000). It is feared that some individuals may pressurize terminally ill patients to seek for euthanasia unwillingly. Moreover, antagonists to this debate fear that medics may go against the will of the patients in executing euthanasia, since regulations may give them overall mandate of making vital decisions over the lives of patients.

Euthanasia and Religion

From a religious perspective, euthanasia is viewed to as unethical practice because it seems to compromise religious doctrines especially those which are concerned with life and death (Kimuyu, 2017).

Christians hold that birth and death constitutes the fundamental life processes that were created by God, and they are ought to be respected because they are sacred. They further claim that life is a sacred gift from God which has to be treated with dignity (Shiflett & Carroll, 2002). Muslims claim that life is a sacred gift from Allah and; therefore, human beings do not have any right to decide over birth and death. As such, assisted suicide appears to fall out of the Islamic doctrines. Moreover, Hindus view euthanasia as social vice that may compromise the Karma of patients and medics. In general, the world's popular religions are against euthanasia because it contravenes the fundamental religious doctrines.

Legislation on Euthanasia

Legislations over euthanasia issue have not yet been put in place in most countries, but there are possible approaches that may lead to universal legitimization or prohibition of euthanasia (Kimuyu, 2018). In the United Kingdom, some legislators have been making relentless attempts to formulate a legal Act that may help to shed light over euthanasia practice. The Assisted Dying Bill of 2006 sought to allow terminally ill patients to receive dying assistance through euthanasia. This bill was proposed by Lord Joffe, but the House of Lords have temporarily blocked it until a comprehensive evaluation is done. Lord Jeffe's bill preceded the Right-to-Die Bill that evoked unprecedented controversy across the U.K with religious leaders raising their voices over the issue.

In contrast, euthanasia had been in practice, in Holland, since 2001. Netherlands is the only country in the world, which has a legal framework that defines euthanasia through the Dutch Law. Moreover, legalization of euthanasia seems to have been enhanced by the Dignity Act of 1994, which legalized assisted suicide.

Conclusion

Conclusively, euthanasia is an old-age practice that emerged among the Ancient Greeks, and it has become widespread in the modern world. This could be probably the reason as to why the Dutch incorporated euthanasia in their constitution.

Euthanasia, which simply meant "easy death", according to the Greeks, has been incorporated in the medical field as part of treatment approaches. However, the varied forms of euthanasia encompass diverse ethical issues. Some social groups in the society view euthanasia as a considerable violation of moral values. Some of these groups include religious leaders and some legislators. On the other hand, proponents of euthanasia view it as a reliable medical approach that helps to reduce agony to terminally ill patients.

However, the untimely dilemma over euthanasia issue has been caused by the unprecedented lack of universality in the legal framework of most countries in the world. Therefore, legal approaches seem to be the only reliable solution to the widespread debate.

References

Bowie, B., & Bowie, R. (2004). *Ethical Studies*. Nashville, TN: Nelson Thornes.

Busè, A. (2008). *Euthanasia- An Overview about Forms, Differences and Difficulties*. Munich, Germany: GRIN Verlag.

Dobson, K., & Galbraith, K. (2000). The Role of the Psychologist in Determining Competence for Assisted Suicide/euthanasia in the Terminally Ill. *Canadian Psychology, 41*, 7-23.

Foley, K., & Hendin, H. (2002). *The Case against Assisted Suicide: For the Right to End-Of-Life Care*. Baltimore, MD: JHU Press.

Frost, M. (n.d). *The Ethics of Euthanasia*. Retrieved from http://www.martinfrost.ws/htmlfiles/scottish_anatomy/euthanasia_ethics.html

Keown, J. (2002). *Euthanasia, Ethics and Public Policy: An Argument against Legalization*. Cambridge, UK: University Press.

Kimuyu, P. (2017). *The Euthanasia Debate: Major Arguments and Religious Perspectives*. Munich, Germany: GRIN Verlag. Retrieved from https://www.grin.com/document/411985

Kimuyu, P. (2018). *Ethics of Physician Assisted Suicide*. Munich, Germany: GRIN Verlag, https://www.grin.com/document/387500

Nicholson, R. (2000). No Painless Death yet for European Euthanasia Debate. *The Hastings Center Report, 30*, 3-16.

Shiflett, D., & Carroll, V. (2002). *Christianity on Trial: Arguments against Anti-Religious Bigotry*, San Francisco, CA: Encounter Books.

YOUR KNOWLEDGE HAS VALUE

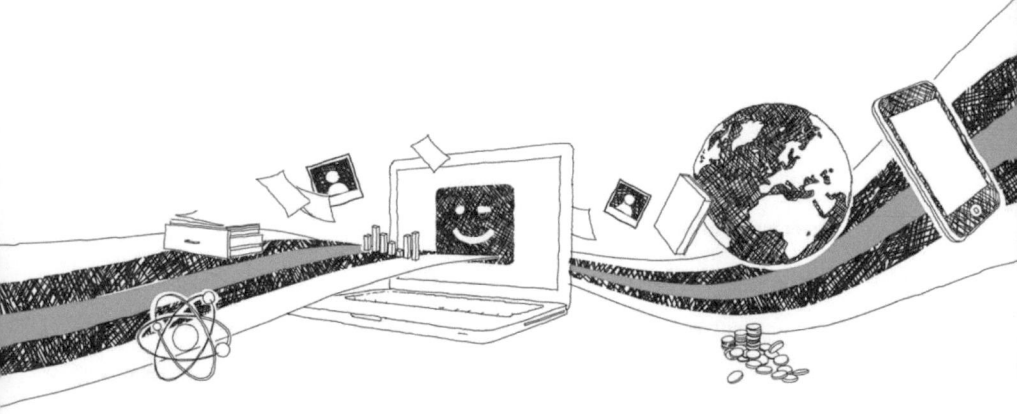

- We will publish your bachelor's and master's thesis, essays and papers

- Your own eBook and book - sold worldwide in all relevant shops

- Earn money with each sale

Upload your text at www.GRIN.com
and publish for free

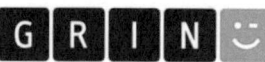